If Hair Could Talk

A Soul-Stirring Journey Through Beauty,
Identity & Purpose

Tim Johnson

Copyright © 2025 Tim Johnson All rights reserved

The characters and events portrayed in this book are fictitious. Any similarity to real persons, living or dead, is coincidental and not intended by the author.

No part of this book may be reproduced, or stored in a retrieval system, or transmitted in any form or by any means, electronic, mechanical, photocopying, recording, or otherwise, without express written permission of the publisher.

ISBN-13: 979-8-9994403-0-3

Printed in the United States of America

If Hair Could Talk is more than a book.

It's an experience.

A movement.

A legacy in motion.

                    –Tim Johnson

Table of Contents

Foreword V

Introduction VII

Disclaimer IX

Chapter One 1

Chapter Two 6

Chapter Three 14

Chapter Four 22

Chapter Five 29

Chapter Six 33

Acknowledgments 42

Your Next Chapter Starts Here 44

About the Author 45

Foreword

In my four decades behind the chair, working with celebrities, dignitaries, and everyday kings, I've learned that what happens in a barber's chair is never just about hair. It's about presence. Connection. Healing. And every now and then, someone comes along who doesn't just master the craft but redefines it. That someone is Tim Johnson.

I've known Tim for over 15 years, watched him on stage. Observed him behind the chair. Witnessed him speak life into broken people all through the language of hair. And I say language because to Tim, hair doesn't just sit silently on the head. It speaks. Loudly.

He once said to me, "If someone's hair is dry, brittle, or lifeless, it's not always about the product. Sometimes, it's grief. Sometimes, it's burnout. Sometimes, it's trauma that hasn't found a voice yet." That shook me. And over the years, I've seen him prove that over and over again. Eight times out of ten, he can tell what someone is carrying just by touching their hair.

That's not just skill. That's spiritual sensitivity. That's divine discernment. And that's what makes Tim a rare and needed voice in this industry. He doesn't just give you a style, he gives you restoration, a reset. Clients walk into his space burdened by life and leave with more than a finished look; they leave lighter, healed, and seen.

See, I've long believed that 95% of this industry is how we make people feel. The haircut is just 5%. But Tim takes that belief and builds a movement around it. He creates a sacred space. A sanctuary. And through this book, he's inviting you to do the same.

If Hair Could Talk is not a gimmick. It's a revelation. It's a blueprint for every barber, stylist, and beauty professional who wants to make an impact, not just income. It's about listening deeper, serving fuller, and leading with heart.

Read every word slowly. Let it settle in your spirit. And the next time you step behind your chair…listen.

Because hair always tells the truth. And when you know how to listen…You become more than a professional. You become a healer.

–DL Master Barber

Introduction

If Hair Could Talk... It would tell the truth we've been avoiding. Let me start by saying this ain't your average book on beauty. This isn't just about hair. It is about the hands that touch it, the hearts that carry it, and the legacy that's braided into every strand. This book is about you—the stylist, the barber, the creative, the visionary, the leader—who's gifted, anointed, called, and may be just a little tired. Perhaps even a little lost. But still hungry for more.

First things, first. I wrote this because I've lived this.

I've stood behind the chair for decades. I've poured into people from every walk of life—mothers, moguls, ministers, millionaires, the broken and the brand new. I've hosted stages, led shows, trained the gifted, and cried with clients who didn't just need a style—they needed a safe place.

And what I discovered is this: hair carries history.

It carries trauma.

It carries triumph.

It carries silence.

It carries strength.

It carries shame, beauty, identity, and purpose.

If hair could talk, it would cry for clarity. Scream for strategy. Warn you about burnout, whisper legacy, and challenge you to rise into who you were born to be.

I need you to understand something as you read this:

You are not just in the beauty business. You are in the transformation business. You carry influence that shift atmospheres. You restore confidence and dignity with your hands—and whether you know it or not, your chair is not just a chair. It is a confessional, a sanctuary, and a throne.

This book will walk you through what most stylists and barbers never get in school: the courage to own your calling, the strategy to master your money, the structure to fuel your growth, the healing to rise from burnout, boldness to build your brand, and a fire for your future.

I'm going to challenge your mindset, confront your patterns, and remind you of the greatness on your life that you may have ignored for too long.

And here's your disclaimer:

After this moment, you will either sleep better than you've ever slept—or you won't sleep at all. Because clarity gives you rest, or it gives you responsibility.

If you're tired of being overlooked, underpaid, burnt out, and boxed in…

If you're ready to step fully into your lane, elevate your brand, honor your gift, and build something eternal, then turn the page.

This is your permission slip to expand, your mirror to see clearly, and your moment to blow up—on purpose.

Let's go.

Blow up, baby.

— Tim Johnson

Disclaimer

(Read This Before You Turn the Page)

Let me be straight with you. This ain't the introduction. And it sure ain't Chapter One.
This is the wake-up bell before the work begins.
Before you dive in, I need to give you a public disclaimer.

This book is about to hit you in one of two ways:

You're either going to lie in bed tonight wide awake, vision racing, trying to figure out how to grab a notebook with one hand and breathe through the excitement with the other because something finally clicked.

Or—you're going to sleep like you haven't in years. Why? Because clarity calms the mind. And this book carries clarity.

In other words, it's going to either ignite you or ground you. Either way, you're going to be changed.

Now, let's be real. This is not a how-to book. It is an internal jolt you didn't know you needed. It's not here to impress you with fancy strategies or step-by-step formulas. It's here to call something out of you, remind you of what you've been sleeping on, and disrupt the lie that says, "One day."

Consider yourself warned: this book is not casual, or your average read. It's a wake-up call and business blueprint for the gifted who got stuck. It's a mindset makeover for the tired visionary who's been playing small and calling it humility.

Here's what I've seen—and I've seen it over and over again.

Most people don't need more advice. They need permission. Yes, permission. Permission to build and finally go get what's already been calling them. They don't need motivation; they need activation.

I'm telling you right now, if you've ever felt like there's more in you—this is your moment.

If you've ever been paralyzed between dreaming and doing—this is the interruption you prayed for but didn't recognize coming.

Now listen—activation is one thing. Execution is another.

Most people get stirred up, only to have life tap them on the shoulder with some distraction: a text, a bill, a bad mood, a phone call… and boom, vision paused.

This book is here to slap that cycle clean out your hands. It's where the mindset shift kicks in. You've been activated. Now you've got to choose. What will your choice be? Will you respect this moment enough to move like it matters?

Lastly, this book is your call to move differently. To see yourself as you really are and stop apologizing for the part of you that's gifted, called, and ready. Note to self, you're not becoming someone else. You're becoming the version of you that's been buried under doubt, duty, and delay. When you finally accept that, you'll walk through the door and into the room.

And once you're in that room, you'll realize that you've belonged here the whole time. You just needed someone to flip the light switch.

This is your moment. Not the soft, "maybe-one-day" moment…but the this-is-it moment.

I charge you to read this book slowly. Highlight what hits. Take a break if you need to—but come back. Because once you start seeing what's possible, you'll never want to shrink back to small talk, small dreams, or small faith again.

Now, turn the page and let your journey begin.

Chapter One

If Hair Could Talk, It Would Tell the Truth

Theme: Identity, Calling, and the Spiritual Weight of Beauty

Let's get this out of the way:

People lie.

Hair doesn't.

You can dress yourself up. Beat your face to the gods. Throw on red bottoms and walk like you've got it all together.

But if your hair could talk—it would whisper the truth.

And if you know how to listen, it's already telling it.

A woman can walk in styled head-to-toe, but the moment she takes a seat, I can see what's really going on. If her hair is neglected, dry, worn out, or simply hidden away—something deeper is speaking.

Now hear me: this ain't about judging anyone. This is about decoding the truth your crown has been carrying.

Some of the women who sit in my chair have the healthiest hair they've ever had—strong, full, thick—but they don't touch it. They don't celebrate it. They don't style it.

Why?

Because deep down, they don't believe it's enough. They don't see their hair as valuable. They've never been taught to honor what they already have. That's identity.

Somewhere between comparison, criticism, and conditioning, they started believing their hair had to be something it wasn't in order to be beautiful, professional, accepted—or simply worthy. When that lie takes root, their crown becomes the first thing to suffer.

That's where I come in.

I work in a private, two-chair studio suite. And I call it "my space" for a reason.

It's more than a salon—it's a sanctuary. The moment a woman walks in, the atmosphere goes to work on her spirit. It's calm, centered, and open. There's a stillness you can feel before you even hear a word.

And the truth is—some women walk in carrying internal chaos. They're running on fumes. Full of noise. Full of shame. And then suddenly... they're surrounded by peace. There's a fragrance in the room you can smell... but also one you can feel. I call that the atmospheric fragrance of acceptance. Because in my chair, you don't have to perform. You don't have to prove, you just have to show up. That's where transformation begins.

When she sits down, I drape her. And when I drape her, I'm not just covering her clothes—I'm clearing the noise. Now we're working from the neck up, a blank canvas. Then we face the mirror. And when I say "we," I mean we. She doesn't face it alone. I stand beside her. And I watch—not just her hair, but her eyes. If she looks down... if she avoids her own reflection... I know. There's shame there. There's pain. There's a woman who's been judged, abandoned, overlooked, or just completely forgotten about herself.

That's what I call hair shame. And listen, hair shame isn't about appearance. It's about everything that's happened above the shoulders, everything life has dumped into her mind, her confidence, her self-image.

Was she told she'd never be good enough? Did she survive heartbreak, betrayal, or divorce? Is she carrying a business, a family, a broken dream, or just herself?

Guess what, hair remembers all of it.

And when she opens up—sometimes without saying a word—that's when I know I'm not just working with strands. I'm working with her story. My chair becomes a confessional.

She begins to speak, not just with her words—but with her presence.

"I over-processed it."

"I ignored it."

"I fried it."

"I just didn't care."

Translation.

"I lost myself."

"I gave up."

"I've been through something, and my hair couldn't hide it."

And that brings me to Meredith.

Meredith is the type of woman whose name you don't forget. Elegant. Sharp. Always on point. A high-performing, self-motivated leader, who balanced family, business, and everything in between like a master conductor—until her marriage blindsided her. Her husband wanted a divorce. And just like that, the rhythm of her world shifted.

She had always worn wigs—beautiful ones, big ones, the kind that made you take notice. But under those wigs, she had disconnected from her own hair. For years, she never touched it, never styled it, never truly saw it. And in many ways, she stopped seeing herself.

About a year before the breakdown, we had talked about making a change. Something bold. A new direction. But it wasn't time. She wasn't ready. Then one day, out of nowhere, I got the message:

"Tim, I think I'm ready."

She came in, slowly removed the wig, and revealed something sacred—herself. To my surprise, her hair was thick, strong, and stunning—salt and pepper, past her shoulders, full of untouched glory. I asked what she had in mind. She looked up and said, "Whatever you think. I want color too."

I went to work—soft caramel browns, warm highlights, a sculpted collar-length bob. Something that felt elegant, refined, but fresh. When I turned her to the mirror, she wept. Not because she looked good, she always had. But because for the first time in years… she looked like herself.

No hiding. No armor. Just Meredith, reintroduced.

That's the power of alignment. When identity catches up to image—and everything inside says, "Yes… This is me."

So now, let me speak directly to stylists, barbers, and beauty professionals:

This chapter is your invitation—and your challenge. Start listening to more than just your clients' words. Listen to what they're bringing into your chair. Listen to what their hair is saying—about their confidence, their grief, their transition, their hope.

Don't just listen. Hear. Tune your ear, tune your heart, and tune your approach.

Ask yourself:

How do I want them to feel when they sit down in my chair?

What kind of experience am I creating for them—right now, and going forward?

Because it's more than freestyle, it's more than a crisp fade or a flawless press. It's about what happens above the shoulders and beneath the surface.

If hair could talk... it would ask you to speak with your hands, your heart, and your gift.

So, I ask you:

Are you styling looks...or stewarding lives?

The difference? I am glad you asked, because that's where the breakthrough lives.

Chapter Two

If Hair Could Talk, It Would Cry for Clarity

Theme: Vision, Structure, and Professional Foundation

Let's stop talking about clients for a minute.

This one's for you—the stylist, the barber, the student, the ambitious creative trying to figure out how to turn a pair of shears into a career and a calling. I want your full attention, because what I'm about to tell you could change everything if you let it.

This chapter is about clarity.

Because let's be real. Most people don't fail because they lack talent. They fail because they're not clear.

And if hair could talk, it would cry out for clarity—loud, raw, and desperate. Not because it needs a perfect curl or the right product, but because it's tired of carrying confusion.

My beginning wasn't perfect. Yours doesn't have to be either.

Let me take you back.

I didn't grow up knowing how to style hair. I wasn't a prodigy. I didn't fall in love with cutting hair at age nine. No, you're looking at a college dropout. A country boy from Raleigh, North Carolina, who could sing but couldn't read a lick of music theory. I was accepted into East Carolina University's music program because of my gift, but my lack of foundation is what got me cut.

My professor told me straight:

"Timothy, you have the gift. But if you don't know the theory, you will not last."

That hit hard. But what really broke me was giving up. I stopped showing up. I lost clarity and quit. But guess what, clarity came next. In a dorm room, with a set of clippers that I had no clue how to use, my boy begged me to cut his hair. I told him no. He begged me again to cut his hair, and I finally said yes. And I jacked him up.

But something clicked.

The very next week, while waiting for my barber, I studied everything. Their posture, their movement, how they held the blade, how they moved the head, how they made the chair spin. And when I went back to campus, I tried again. I got better, word spread, and the next thing I knew, I was the bootleg campus barber, cutting hair for $3 a head, football players and all.

Let that sink in.

The thing that changed my life started as a mistake. But I was present enough to notice the opportunity in it.

The Door to Destiny Sometimes Looks Like Rejection

Eventually, school pushed me out. My GPA was a 0.83, which led to academic probation, and you know the rest. I couldn't go back in the fall.

But failure put me in front of a decision. Curl up in shame or shift. I told my mom I was switching paths, barber school. However, I encountered some opposition, including an over a year waitlist, and nothing close by.

Then I had a conversation with a professional stylist. I told him my dilemma. He said, "Why not go to cosmetology school?" I said, "I don't do women's hair. I don't want that stigma. I don't think stylists make money." And he smiled. Then he showed me his numbers. Suddenly, I wasn't laughing anymore. I was listening. That man became my mentor. He walked me into my next chapter. I enrolled. I showed up. And after school, I reported straight to his salon. Shampooing. Running errands. Watching. Learning.

He told me something critical. "Don't tell your instructors how much you're learning with me. Just show up like a blank canvas and absorb." So that's what I did. I was learning in the classroom—and I was learning about real life in the salon. In the classroom, I stayed locked in—learning theory, state board prep, and the foundational knowledge every professional needs. But in the salon, I was soaking up the stuff no textbook could teach—client behavior, salon flow, how to carry myself, how to sell, and how to really serve people. It was a masterclass in humility and hustle. I was building my future from both sides: the books and the experience. That head start became my competitive edge. And that's what I want for you.

The Reason You Feel Invisible Has Nothing to Do with Your Skill

If you feel invisible right now in your career, it's not because you're not good enough. It's because you haven't been seen. And sometimes, that's because you haven't discovered yourself yet.

Let's be brutally honest.

If you've been in the industry 1–2 years and still feel stuck, it's not because of "bad luck." It's because you've never been trained how to position your greatness. You're winging it. You're freestyling your future.

Talent without direction is noise. So, let's clean up the noise.

Here's the formula:

- Get clear on your skill.
- Get clear on your system.
- Get clear on your story.
- Get clear on your pricing.
- Get clear on your identity.

You are not here to just "do hair." You are here to deliver an experience, define a standard, and dominate your lane.

Systems Are Not Optional. They Are Survival.

Let's talk business.

What's your onboarding system? How do clients find you? What happens when they land on your page?

What kind of first impressions are you making?

Do you have a QR code? A lead magnet? A referral incentive?

Do they book appointments through DMs or through an actual platform that makes it seamless?

Once they're in your chair—what's their experience?

Are you present? Are you educated? Are you communicating?

When they leave, do they want to come back because of the hair—or because of how you made them feel?

Whew, I know that is a lot.

If you don't know how to answer these questions, don't panic.

Just get serious.

Because the pros aren't better than you, they're just more prepared than you.

Pricing Panic Kills Careers

Let's go here.

Some of y'all are charging $45 for a $150 experience. Others are charging $150 for a $45 result.

Both are dangerous.

You cannot afford to play guessing games with your price list. Study your market. Study your value. Study your results—price for impact, not just income. When your pricing lacks strategy, it can either drain your spirit or damage your reputation. Confidence comes from clarity. Know what you're worth, then charge like it.

Pricing panic kills careers because it keeps you second-guessing your value, doubting your skill, and chasing validation instead of building vision. Back-and-forth, that's what burns you out and breaks trust with your clients.

This is where a mentor's impact takes form, creating a lifeline. A mentor brings stability where there's confusion. They help you align your price with your promise, so you're not just hoping you're worth it, you know you are.

You don't need another discount; you need direction.

And if you don't know what to charge, that's the signal you need a mentor, not a new logo.

Client Cycles Are Real—But Your Confidence Shouldn't Waver

Clients rotate. Some will stay loyal for years. Others will disappear. It's life. But when your client schedule shifts, don't spiral. Don't question your gift. Double down on your systems.

Keep marketing. Keep refining. Keep showing up.

When it feels slow, build stronger. When it feels fast, scale smarter. This means using quiet seasons to upgrade your client experience, content, and strategy. You're not just waiting, you're preparing. And when business picks up, don't just survive the rush—optimize it, delegate, raise your standards, and move with intention. Every season has a purpose if you manage it wisely.

Which leads me to the next thing. Your confidence cannot live in your calendar. It has to live in your clarity.

Build an Experience That Speaks

Let me say this as loudly and clearly as possible.

If people are only coming to you for a "style," you've already lost.

They should be coming to you for how you make them feel when they sit in your chair, a connection.

Ask yourself, What's your atmosphere like? What's your fragrance? What's your sound?

What's your presence? Are you someone they can relax with? Are you creating a space where people can exhale?

When you ask yourself these questions, you're unlocking the blueprint for a next-level client experience. It's not just about the service; it's about the soul of your space. When clients feel seen, safe, and valued, they don't just come back; they bring others. This is how loyalty is built. This is how legacy is born. You're not just styling hair... you're shaping atmosphere, identity, and emotional connection. That's what they'll remember long after the curls fall.

Rest assured, this experience is a luxury. Not marble countertops. Not overpriced bundles. It's intentional energy. Elevated care. It's real results.

Your Challenge

I challenge you—right now—to get clear.

Not next month. Not after you "get a few more followers." Now.

Clarity starts on paper before it shows up in your life. This isn't just a reflection exercise; it's your turning point. Because the moment you define it, you start becoming it.

Answer these questions. And don't just think about them, write them down. When you write it, you activate it.

Who are you?

What do you do better than anyone else?

What kind of experience do you want to be known for?

Next, I want you to build your system. Own your sound. And commit to never showing up confused again. Because when clarity hits, confusion dies, comparison fades, and compensation explodes.

If hair could talk…It would say, "Let's finally build this right, with clarity."

Chapter Three

If Hair Could Talk, It Would Scream for Strategy

Theme: Branding with Identity, Building Wealth with Intention, Becoming Unforgettable in Your Lane

Let me tell you something straight off.

You can't cut your way to freedom. You can't curl your way to wealth. And you sure can't style your way to purpose—unless you start thinking like a brand.

My career didn't shift because I was just good behind the chair. It turned the day I realized I was the brand—not just my business name, not just my logo, not even my salon, but me. I was the business. I was the system.

If you don't see yourself as a brand, you'll only ever see yourself as a hustle. You'll crank out curls, bangs, fades, braids—for what? A few dollars and sore feet. The moment you begin to see yourself differently and claim your identity as a walking brand, you activate something powerful. Now, you're no longer just styling hair—you're building a legacy. And that's where I want you to be.

Let me break it down for you.

If your salon is named *Sensational Hair*, and people only recognize you as "the lady from Sensational Hair," then you're invisible. But if you've branded yourself correctly, they'll say, "Hey, that's Sharon—she owns Sensational Hair."

See the difference.

Branding is more than a logo. It's how you move. It's the fragrance of how your business feels. It's the vibe, the atmosphere, the experience. Your brand is your identity in motion.

Build Wealth with Intention

Here's a harsh truth: If you don't build wealth on purpose, you'll spend your whole life reacting.

There was a time I had to look myself in the mirror and say, "I don't want to be standing behind this chair for the rest of my life."

That realization forced me to think differently. I had to turn my brand into a machine, a vehicle that generated wealth even when I wasn't behind the chair. That's when the game changed.

I started doing more than hair. I began participating in industry events, and then I started speaking. Later, I launched my own product line. I even built my own shows and educational experiences. Each move was intentional, adding a new income stream. Most importantly, each move brought me back more freedom.

Let me share with you what freedom looks like. It looks like your product line making just as much or more than you make in the salon. It looks like one event paying your rent, covering your bills, and still leaving you with profit. It means your time is no longer tied to a client schedule but to your calling.

I said all of that to say, you can't just hustle your way to success. You've got to design it, strategize it, and own every move you make.

Multiple Irons in the Same Fire

Have you ever heard the saying "don't be a jack of all trades"?

Let me flip that for you. Be the master of your one trade. Then find multiple ways to dominate it.

If you do hair, that's great.

Now ask yourself, what else can I create from this one trade?

Bonus—I'll give you several:

- A product line
- A course
- A retreat or mastermind
- An e-book or journal
- An event, tour, or platform show

Now it's your turn. What's on your list? What ideas have been sitting in your spirit, waiting to be activated? Write them down. Speak them out loud. Pray over them. Build from them. The more ways your gift can work for you, the less you'll have to hustle to prove it.

Stack your irons in the same fire and then turn up the heat.

Work Gets Work: Master the Client Journey

One of my foundational principles is this: Work gets work.

Too many stylists and barbers are sitting at home waiting for the phone to ring, scrolling through social media, wondering why the clients aren't coming. Let me tell you something—if you're not in motion, neither is your money.

When I first started, I had to learn this the hard way. I called my mentor and asked him to call me if someone walked in needing a stylist. You know what he said?

"Get off your butt and come to work. This business doesn't grow in your living room."

That checked me real quick.

If your book isn't full, your job isn't to chill—it's to build. Build by creating content, calling past clients, and doing outreach. Use this time to strategize your next move. Get creative, bring in models, run promotions. Be sure to audit what's working and what's not because everything you do in the quiet season prepares you for momentum. And that momentum is the fuel that powers the full client journey.

This is what it means to master the client's journey from the first point of contact to repeat loyal customers.

Let's go a little further. Ask yourself, what's your onboarding process? How do people find you? Do they get ignored when they call or text you? Are you missing out on business opportunities because you won't answer the phone?

Fix it.

This generation of consumers is instant. If they don't feel seen, they move on. Your voicemail, your DMs, your email, your site—all of it should scream, "I'm professional. I'm ready. And I'm worth your time."

From booking to blowout, your brand should be flawless.

Social Media Isn't Marketing, It's Exposure

Let's be real for a second. Social media ain't marketing. It's exposure. That's it.

Instagram, Facebook, TikTok, LinkedIn — they're all windows. People can peek in, get curious, and feel your energy. But don't confuse that with a strategy. Social media is where they find you, not where they hire you.

You post to stay visible. You show your results. You let people catch your rhythm. But the real work happens off the app — in your systems, your follow-up, your retention, and your client journey.

Use social media to start the conversation, not to run your business. Expose your excellence, then guide people to your real house: your booking link, your email list, your offers, your world.

This is not about going viral. This is about being valuable consistently. This is how exposure becomes income. It's how followers become clients.

Social media is spiritual—people post what they want you to believe. But real marketing is what you build outside the scroll.

Let's be clear, marketing is more than content. It's a connection. It's consistency. It's how people experience you when the phone is down and the feed is quiet.

So let me ask you:

Are you positioned in real life the way you appear online?

Is your presence as strong in the streets as it is in your Stories on social media?

Do you have a QR code that leads to a full breakdown of your brand?

Do you carry digital business cards that make you easy to remember?

Do you show up at community events and industry spaces where your people are already gathered?

If the answer is "not yet," now's the time to tighten it up. Your brand deserves more than a post— it deserves presence. It's how people experience you. People don't just want to see your work. They want to feel your energy.

You are your billboard, and every interaction is a commercial for your brand.

The Product Line: Nobody's Buying Because You're Not Selling

Let's talk facts.

In 2020, when the world shut down, I couldn't rely on my salon. My team couldn't come in. I couldn't serve clients. But the bills didn't shut down. So, what did I do? I pivoted.

I launched Tim Johnson Systems—starting with a product I had already developed: It's Butta Baby, a multi-use butter for hair, beard, and body. I had the chemist. I had the formula. I had the packaging. But I was sitting on it.

Why? Impostor syndrome.

I had helped other brands build empires, but I wasn't pushing my own. I had an entire line but wasn't selling it.

Here's the truth: if you've got a product and you're not selling, it's not because people don't want it—it's because you haven't committed. That's right, you have not committed to promoting it. Committed to packaging it right or committed to believing in it the same way you believe in everybody else's. Your product can't speak until you do. And the world won't buy in until you show up.

I'm challenging you right now to push your product. Promote your service and sell what you've been hiding. In doing so, make sure you show up with fire.

The Six-Figure Salon Without Burnout

I had a six-figure salon, but I was working myself into the ground—15 to 20 clients a day, 6 days a week, falling asleep behind the wheel. That's not wealth. That's wage slavery in disguise.

The quarantine forced me to pause. And I realized I had built a machine that was breaking me. Something had to change. So, I reinvented it.

Now, I work by appointment only. I run multiple income streams. I coach, speak, create, and rest—on my terms. Six figures is great, but freedom is better.

Let me leave you with this. You are not just a stylist. You are not just a barber. You are not just a beauty professional. You are a brand. You are a system. You are a movement.

I challenge you to build it with purpose, price it with confidence, promote it with fire, and protect your peace while doing it.

Because if hair could talk, it would shout, "Get paid on purpose—and don't burn out doing it."

Chapter Four

If Hair Could Talk, It Would Warn You

Theme: Mental Health, Spiritual Alignment, and Leadership Integrity

Let me talk to you straight.

If hair could talk… it wouldn't just whisper. It wouldn't just tell the truth. By now, it would be screaming. Screaming at the stylist who's on her feet 12 hours a day, smiling through the pain. Screaming at the barber who's always booked but battling depression in silence. Screaming at the beautypreneur whose brand is booming but their soul is running on empty.

This chapter is not for the faint of heart. It's for the one who looks successful on paper but is crumbling in private. It's for the future stylist just entering the game, wide-eyed and hopeful. And it's for the vet who's tired, worn out, and wondering if the passion can ever come back.

I wrote this for YOU.

Because I lived this. I know what it feels like to pour from an empty cup. To be celebrated on the outside while silently breaking on the inside. To lead with excellence while quietly praying for strength just to make it through the day.

I didn't write this chapter to impress you—I wrote it to *rescue* you. Because no one told us that purpose could be heavy. That passion could burn us out. But know this, healing is possible, and alignment is available. This chapter is your permission to pause, to be honest with yourself, and to come back into agreement with the version of you God actually called—not the one you've been performing as.

Burnout Is Not Branding

Let's kill the myth right now. Burnout is not a badge of honor. It is not proof of greatness, and it sure is not part of your brand.

I learned this the hard way.

Straight out of cosmetology school, I exploded. I had mentorship, vision, and hunger. I was on fire—and the industry felt it. In my first week out, I earned over $860. Within three months, I was averaging $1,500 a week in 1989.

But no one warned me what success without balance costs. No one told me what unchecked ambition will rob you of. No one pulled me aside and said, "Tim, you're about to build a business that might bury you."

I stood on my feet for years. Long days. No boundaries. No breaks. I was delivering beauty—but inside, I was breaking. And you know the worst part? My clients were happy. They were raving. But I knew… I wasn't giving my best.

I'd see pictures later and feel the guilt—because while they loved it, I knew I was slacking. Not from lack of skill but from lack of rest. Lack of soul-care. Lack of alignment.

Success at the cost of your peace is not success. It's slavery dressed up in applause.

You're Overbooked and Underfed

Being overbooked might impress your followers. But your spirit knows the truth: you're starving. You can't feed the world and forget to feed yourself.

We live in a time where "booked and busy" is the goal—but let me warn you; "booked and bitter" is where many end up.

All money isn't good money. Not all clients are meant to sit in your chair. And just because you can fit another appointment in doesn't mean you should. Being overbooked without boundaries leads to exhaustion, resentment, sloppy work, and yes—burnout that breaks your body and your brilliance.

You're underfed spiritually. No stillness. No silence. No time to hear God. No time to breathe. And if you're not hearing God, you're just grinding…on your own power.

The Salon, The Stress, and The Spirit

Let's be clear, the salon is not your sanctuary. It's not your refuge. It is your workplace. It must work for you—not the other way around.

If you've turned your identity into your chair, you're in danger. The salon is a business, not a god. And when you idolize the grind, you invite the curse of depletion.

Stress is what happens when you try to do in your own power what only God can sustain. It'll sneak up on you—behind the wheel, behind the chair, behind the smile. I've fallen asleep at stoplights. I've nodded off in my own salon, waking up hours later on the floor. I've worked myself into headaches, high blood pressure, weight gain, and spiritual dryness.

And for what?

A booked schedule with no boundaries will have your body breaking down and your brand falling apart.

Here's the truth: rest is spiritual. Stillness is strategy. Silence is where the next level downloads.

Sleep. Rest. Relaxation.

There's a difference between sleep, rest, and relaxation. And you need all three. Sleep is what keeps your body alive. Rest is what renews your soul. Relaxation is what reconnects you to yourself.

You cannot pour out power if you're never plugged in.

So, ask yourself:

Do you have a nightly routine that protects your peace? Do you create space in your week to breathe—not just sleep, but rest? Do you intentionally choose joy? Laughter? Stillness? Movement? Unplugging?

Most importantly, are you prioritizing your peace? Because if you don't prioritize your peace, your body will force you to.

How to Stay Clean in a Dirty Industry

Let's not act like this industry is all glitz and glam. There's a dark side. There's gossip. Manipulation. Stealing clients. Undercutting and straight-up shade. And if you're not grounded spiritually, emotionally, and professionally—you'll get swept up in it without even realizing it.

But here's the truth: just because mess is around you doesn't mean it has to get in you. You've got to decide early who you're going to be. Operate with honor. Speak life, not lies. Protect your reputation like it's your credit—because in this industry, it is. Stay prayed up. Keep your head down. Do excellent work. And when you rise, rise clean. This industry doesn't need more drama. It needs more light.

Don't let the dirt in the industry pull you down. Stay clean. Stay honorable.

One of my mentors taught me early that when you see someone with a beautiful style, compliment the work even if you didn't do it. Say, "whoever did your hair, they did a great job." You don't have to cut someone else down to build yourself up. There are enough heads out here for all of us. Enough gifts. Enough glory. Enough ground.

Lead with integrity. Your hands will speak long before your mouth ever opens.

Leadership vs. Lordship

Let me share a hard truth with you.

One of my early mentors was brilliant—but toxic. He had a gift, but his tongue. Sharp. Cutting. Cruel. One day, I was shampooing a young girl with tightly coiled hair. I didn't know how to manage it. I needed help. And instead of training me, he humiliated me. Called me stupid, loudly and publicly.

That moment could have broken me. Instead, I walked away and found better leadership. Leadership that corrects without condemning. That teaches without tearing down. If you're in a leadership position, don't forget that people are fragile, but they're also full of fire. It's your job to coach, not crush. To lift, not lord. To correct in love, not dominate with ego.

Great leaders multiply greatness in others. Not fear.

Final Word: Take Care of You

Let me say this clearly. Your chair is not your identity, and your grind is not your god.

Take care of your mental health.

Get a therapist if you need to. That's not weakness—it's wisdom. Make time for your family, your healing, your hobbies, your joy. Because when YOU are whole, your work will reflect it. But if you're broken, your business will break too.

I challenge you to do the following:

- Pause before you overbook.
- Listen before you prescribe.
- Discern before you design.
- Protect your peace like your legacy depends on it—because it does.

Don't be the stylist who gets to the top and loses their soul on the way.

If hair could talk, it would warn you and say, take care of YOU.

And if you're willing to listen… you'll realize it's not just about beauty. It's about becoming.

Chapter Five

If Hair Could Talk, It Would Whisper Legacy

Theme: Generational Wealth, Industry Impact, and Kingdom Calling

If hair could talk, it wouldn't just shout trends or scream success. No—it would whisper legacy. Not the loud, fleeting kind of success that burns hot and fizzles out, but the kind that speaks in generations. The kind that leaves a residue of excellence in every salon, every client story, every seed planted. This chapter is about going beyond the chair. It's about impact that outlives your hands. It's about building legacy.

From Chair to Coach to CEO

My journey started just like yours, behind the chair. I was a young man with clippers in one hand, a dream in the other, and no idea just how far this industry would take me. What started as a skill quickly became a lifestyle. And that lifestyle became leadership. But it didn't stop there.

At some point, my chair became more than a place of service—it became a sacred platform. I wasn't just cutting hair. I was hearing confessions and giving advice. I was offering prayer, building trust, and speaking life. Every appointment was part therapy, part transformation.

Eventually, people stopped asking just for a trim—they started asking for strategy. How did I build this business?

How did I stay relevant? How did I stay booked, balanced, and in my bag without burning out? And just like that, I realized I wasn't just a stylist. I had become a coach.

From there, the calling grew louder. I wasn't just coaching individuals—I was launching companies and hosting shows. I was creating educational systems and building platforms that outlived the appointments. I became a CEO not because I wanted a title, but because I had to take ownership of what God was doing through me.

And now... my job is legacy. Period.

Train Don't Just Teach

There's a difference between teaching and training. Teaching fills heads. Training builds hands, hearts, and habits. Most educators in this industry provide information but rarely demand transformation. That stops now.

My goal is to train the next generation to move with purpose. Your stance, your touch, your silence, your speed—it all speaks.

Ask yourself:

Are you confident or chaotic? Are you intentional or insecure? Are you building something or barely holding it together?

Teaching is about knowledge. Training is about preparation. And preparation is the seed of legacy.

Build With an Exit Strategy

Let me talk to the grown folks for a minute. What's your exit strategy? Or are you just hoping to stand behind that chair until your knees give out and your back quits?

Legacy thinkers build now for what they can't do later. I've been in this game for 30+ years. But I'm not just still here—I'm thriving in new rooms. Not because I'm lucky, but because I built systems. Streams. Brands. Strategies.

You cannot retire on passion alone. You need purpose and a plan. This industry isn't just about today's bag—it's about building income that lasts even when your hands no longer can.

Blow Up, Baby: The Call to Build Bigger

"Blow up, baby" is more than a catchphrase. It's a commandment.

Every time I see someone discover the gift they've been ignoring, I say it. Every time I coach a stylist out of survival mode and into strategy, I say it. Every time a student finally realizes that their creativity isn't just art—it's authority, I say it.

You were not created to be average. You were born to blow up in purpose, in profit, and in power. You don't have to be the best in the world, but you'd better become the best in your lane. You don't have to take everyone's spot, just take your place. And when you find it, own it. Scale it. Build on it and pass it on.

If hair could talk, it would say, "I carried more than style, I carried legacy. I was shaped by hands that healed. I held the imprint of vision, the residue of faith, and the echo of excellence passed down. I wasn't just a look…I was a lineage."

The Legacy Challenge

Here's my challenge to you:

1. Build with your name in mind, put your children's children in your heart. Don't just grind for now, invest in tomorrow.

2. Find your lane and dig a trench so deep in it that you could never be forgotten. Be the go-to. The one whose name rings out in the room, even when you're not there.

3. Become the kind of stylist or barber that whispers legacy with every appointment. Let your presence heal and your hands restore. Let your work outlive you.

Remember, God is using you to establish influence and dominion through the gifts in your hands. This isn't just hair—it's harvest.

Now, go BLOW UP BABY!

Chapter Six

If Hair Could Talk, It Would Say This Is Not the End

Theme: Completion, Commissioning, and the Courage to Build What's Next

Let's pause.

Take a breath.

Let the weight of everything you've just read settle in your spirit. Let it settle in, not heavy like a burden—but weighty like purpose. Let it settle in like destiny sitting upright and waiting on your next move.

This is the final chapter, but it's not a period. It's a pivot. A holy turn toward your future. Because now that you know what you know, you can't unknow it. You've heard the whispers of identity and faced the mirror of truth. You've watched clarity turn into strategy, stared burnout in the face, and found your boundaries.

Not only that, you've awakened the voice of legacy that had been buried beneath self-doubt and exhaustion. You didn't just read this book. You confronted your reflection and made peace with the process. You stood in the presence of truth, and you didn't flinch.

This book was never about how to flat iron or fade. It was about the real work. It was about the heart behind the hands, and the vision behind the business. And let's not forget the weight behind the crown or the anointing behind the appointment.

You see, hair has always told the truth. But now... you've learned how to hear it. Now you understand how to translate image into impact. Now, you know you weren't just building a clientele, you were building a legacy.

Let me say this clearly. Your gift is not random. Your ability to transform is not accidental. And your chair is not just a business—it's an altar. A place where brokenness meets beauty and confusion meets clarity. A place where masks come off and identity is restored.

And whether you realized it or not, this book was your ordination. It was your moment of being pulled aside from the noise, be told the truth about yourself, and remember the weight of your influence. It was your moment to recommit to a level of integrity, innovation, and impact that this world can't ignore.

So, let me ask you straight.

Now what?

Now that your heart is stirred, your mind is renewed, and your eyes are opened, what will you do with what you now know?

Will you return to business as usual, or will you return with fire? Will you offer another cut, or will you start offering transformation? Will you keep "freestyling," or will you build something so sharp, so structured, so on purpose—that hell itself will have to back up when you walk in the room?

I am not done. There is more. Will you finally charge what you're worth—not just in price, but in presence? Will you finally treat your brand like a business, not just a hustle? Will you finally invest in the coach, the class, the course, the system that will take you from "busy" to bankable?

Because let me remind you, the world is full of stylists, but very few visionaries. The world has salons, but very few sanctuaries. The world has plenty of trends, but what we need are truth tellers. Gifted, grounded leaders who carry healing in their hands, structure in their systems, and a message in their mirror.

This is your moment. The moment where you stop waiting on permission—and start walking in power. The moment you stop playing small because others aren't dreaming big. The moment you stop comparing your behind-the-scenes to someone else's highlight reel—and build your own movement, your own brand, your own legacy.

You were never meant to blend in. You were born to break the mold. You were designed to disturb the norm. And if you've been waiting on a sign, this is it.

Here we are. Full circle.

You've heard the whispers, the cries, the screams, the warnings, and the legacy. You've walked through every chapter, not just as a reader—but as a witness to your own reflection.

This book was never just about hair. It was about the soul behind the style, the purpose behind the platform, and the divine clarity behind your calling.

From the chair to the stage, from shampoo bowls to boardrooms, we've uncovered what most in this industry avoid. Not because they can't—but because they're afraid of the mirror. Afraid of the truth behind the touch. But you didn't flinch. You leaned in.

You're not just holding shears—you're holding space. You're not just twisting coils or fading lines—you're shifting lives. You're not just booking clients—you're building legacy.

Now let's be clear, none of this works without vision, structure, system, and strategy. Talent alone is loud, but without structure, it fades. What you've been given must be shaped, developed, and multiplied—because what's on you is too valuable to waste on burnout, inconsistency, or comparison.

And if this book did its job, you're no longer invisible. You've been discovered by the one person who needed to find you most—YOU.

You now understand that your chair is a pulpit. Your touch is a ministry. Your strategy is your lifeline, and your story is your superpower. But don't get too comfortable. This was just the activation.

The world doesn't need another stylist. The world needs a transformer. A truth-teller. A brand-builder with integrity. We need leaders whose hands are skilled but whose hearts are aligned. We need you.

So, what now? I'm glad you asked.

Now, you blow up. You create, launch, and multiply with precision. You invest in coaching, mentorship, and mastery—not because you're weak but because you've made peace with the fact that greatness requires guidance. You train others the way you wish someone had trained you.

Take it a step further and expand beyond the chair, beyond the shop, beyond the "likes"—and into purpose, profit, peace, and power. Because legacy doesn't start at retirement. Legacy starts with one decision.

It's the decision to stop shrinking to fit who you were and start rising to become who you were born to be. And when you make that choice—your gift will stand up and clap.

If hair could talk... it would thank you.

It would remind you that you heard what others ignored. That you took the scissors and shaped destiny. You dared to believe your chair was sacred ground and your gift was enough.

So now, I leave you with this.

You were born to build. You were called to change lives. And you were anointed to lead—not just with clippers and combs, but with courage, clarity, and character.

This is not the end. This is the beginning of your next level.

Here's your final challenge:

1. Revisit your chair—not just as a service, but as a stewardship.

2. Rethink your brand—not just as a name, but as a narrative.

3. Redefine your future—not as a fantasy, but as a framework you now have the power to build.

Now, you have strategy. You have structure and a story. And you've got God's breath on your next move.

So, there's nothing left to do but blow up, baby. But this time, not for applause, not for followers or even for validation. This time it is for legacy and impact. It is for the generations watching you. For the women and men who will one day sit in your chair, not even knowing that you almost gave up—until you didn't.

This is your moment. Own it. This is your legacy. Live it. This is your call. Answer it.

If hair could talk, it would say:

"Thank you for hearing me. Now go help someone else hear themselves."

If Hair Could Talk-Chapter Recaps

Disclaimer

The Wake-up Call Before Page One
A bold warning and loving charge: After this moment, you'll either be too ignited to sleep or rest better than you ever have—because clarity has arrived. This book is not a how-to. It's a mirror, a mindset shift, a business blueprint, and a life-altering wake-up call for anyone ready to rise.

Chapter One: If Hair Could Talk, It Would Tell the Truth

Theme: Identity, Calling, and the Spiritual Weight of Beauty

Hair tells on the heart. In this chapter, we explore how neglected hair often reveals neglected identity. Your chair is more than a service spot; it's a sacred space where restoration begins. It includes the powerful story of "Meredith," a woman who finally removed the wig and saw herself again.

Chapter Two: If Hair Could Talk, It Would Cry for Clarity

Theme: Vision, Structure, and Professional Foundation

Before marketing and money, there must be vision. This chapter covers the importance of mentorship, price clarity, intentional service design, and the systems that create long-term transformation for you and your clients.

Chapter Three: If Hair Could Talk, It Would Scream for Strategy

Theme: Branding with Identity, Building Wealth with Intention, Becoming Unforgettable in Your Lane

Success isn't just talent—it's structure. In this chapter we cover what it means to get paid on purpose. Learn to brand with identity, generate multiple streams of income, and avoid burnout by building a life and business that works for you, not against you.

Chapter Four: If Hair Could Talk, It Would Warn You

Theme: Mental Health, Spiritual Alignment, and Leadership Integrity

Leadership without wholeness is dangerous. This chapter dives deep into the private battles of burnout, misalignment, and image management. Your platform must match your personal power. And that starts with healing, boundaries, and truth.

Chapter Five: If Hair Could Talk, It Would Whisper Legacy

Theme: Generational Wealth, Industry Impact, and Kingdom Calling

From chair to coach to CEO—this is the journey of building beyond yourself. Learn the power of influence, the necessity of exit strategies, and the divine assignment of multiplying your gifts. This is about more than hair. This is about history. Yours.

Chapter Six: If Hair Could Talk, It Would Say This Is Not the End

Theme: Completion, Commissioning, and the Courage to Build What's Next

You've been activated. Now, you're accountable. This final chapter ties it all together and launches you forward with boldness, purpose, and power. You don't just have a skill—you have a calling. And legacy is waiting for your name.

Acknowledgments

If Gratitude Could Speak...

This is what it would say.

To my Heavenly Father, my Source, my Strength, my Sustainer. Lord Jesus Christ, thank You for guiding every word, every page, and every moment of this process. This book was born from the quiet whispers of Your Spirit.

To my wife, my partner, my confidant, your unwavering love, friendship, and belief in me are woven into every chapter of my life. Thank you for standing beside me with grace and power.

To my children, Timothy and Taylor, you are my joy and my why. Watching you become who God created you to be is my greatest inspiration.

To my mother, thank you for the love, wisdom, and one-of-a-kind only-child experience that only a phenomenal woman like you could give. Your strength is my foundation.

To my clients, each of you helped me shape this gift. You allowed me to serve with my hands and lead with my heart. Our conversations, transformations, and sacred moments behind the chair are the true pages of this story.

Angela Anderson, your belief in this message pulled this book out of me. Thank you for coaching, pushing, editing, and standing firm in excellence with me. I couldn't have done this without your brilliance.

John Brown, thank you for capturing the essence of who I am through your lens. Your photography has always told the truth with beauty and power.

Shaheran, thank you for translating vision into design. The cover you created doesn't just catch the eye—it tells a story. Phenomenal work.

To everyone who ever prayed for me, spoke life into me, or sat in my chair, you are part of this legacy.

If gratitude could speak... this is what it would sound like.

Your Next Chapter Starts Here

You've read the stories. You've heard the lessons. You've felt the shift. But I don't want our conversation to end here.

I have recorded an exclusive, personal video —a private message from me to you. It's my way of looking you in the eye, speaking life into you, and making sure you leave this book with more than inspiration. I want you to leave with activation.

In this video, I'll share:

- The three truths that have carried me through every season of my career and calling
- The one mindset shift that can immediately change how you see yourself and your future
- A personal declaration over your life — one I believe will mark the start of your next, most powerful chapter

This is not for the masses.
It's for those who made it to this page.
Those who are ready to take what they've read and turn it into something extraordinary.

Watch your personal message now:
www.timjohnsonlive.com

The next level is waiting.
It's time to step into it.

— Tim Johnson

About the Author

Tim Johnson is a transformational beauty industry icon with over three decades of experience behind the chair, on stage, and in the boardroom. As a master stylist, educator, speaker, and spiritual coach, Tim has turned salons into sanctuaries and scissors into instruments of healing. Known for his bold message, powerful presence, and prophetic insight, he challenges stylists, barbers, and entrepreneurs to stop hustling and start building their legacy.

Through his product line, coaching platforms, and groundbreaking tours, Tim empowers professionals to brand with purpose, lead with integrity, and build recession-proof businesses anchored in identity, clarity, and calling.

Tim Johnson isn't just shaping styles…he's awakening purpose, elevating identity, and igniting legacy in every life he touches.

Visit him online at www.timjohnsonlive.com.

www.ingramcontent.com/pod-product-compliance
Lightning Source LLC
Chambersburg PA
CBHW060538030426
42337CB00021B/4327